Keeping your Retina Healthy

A Guide To Retina Conditions, Treatments & Choosing A Retina Specialist

Dr. Amjad Hammad (Dr. Jay)

Saratoga Vitreo-Retinal Ophthalmology
465 Maple Avenue
Unit B
Saratoga Springs, New York 12866

Phone: 518-580-0553
Fax: 518-580-0557

www.SaratogaRetina.com

Dedication

This book is dedicated to my loving and supportive wife Terry, and to my wonderful and dedicated staff Deborah Bowler, Amy Miller, Gina McBride, Colleen Furey, Bridget Demarco and Bobie Schumacher. And most of all the, the thousands of people that have been patients of mine since 1993, in the United States, Jordan and Dubai. For I feel that I have truly learned more from my dear patients than I could possibly give to them. This book is a way for me to make it easier for others to get the treatment and care they deserve as our vision allows us to maintain our quality of life. Every single patient has taught me how deeply and intensely eye pain and vision loss affects their life. How there is an urgent need for answers, a treatment plan and a desire to "feel better again".

Thus I have put together this book for others to overcome their fears and get treatment early. If this book provides one bit of information that gives you peace of mind with regard to any aspect of your eye health, then it will be wildly successful.

When our health fails us we become the most vulnerable and need the most trusted advice. Trusted advice, skilled treatment options and comfort is what we offer you.

Table of Contents

Foreword:

Welcome. My name is Dr. Amjad Hammad. My patients, staff and friends call me Dr. Jay and I am a retina specialist. As a retina specialist I take on some of the most complicated eye problems in the community. As a medical doctor, I understand that our health is one of our biggest fears and losing your vision in particular is an incredibly scary time. Without your vision, it is difficult to maintain your quality of life and continue all of your normal daily activities.

I have dedicated my life to improving people's vision around the world. I take care of a wide variety of retinal conditions from congenital changes and weaknesses to acquired tumors, degenerations (such as age related macular degeneration) and retinal holes/tears and detachments.

We see a lot of patients with retinal complications from diabetes. Every year, almost 2 million new cases of diabetes are diagnosed in people aged 20 years and older and nearly a quarter million children under the age of 20 are affected with the disease.

Diabetes is the leading cause of blindness and nearly 30% of those diagnosed with diabetes will have diabetic retinopathy. Many diabetic eye diseases can be managed if not avoided with proper treatments and blood sugar management. Everyone diagnosed with diabetes should have a thorough eye exam completed as a baseline for follow-on care.

We are partners with our local Northeastern New York Chapter of the Juvenile Diabetes Research Foundation (JDRF) with a mission to help deliver a cure for Type 1 Diabetes.

We believe that if we can provide the proper support early on, we can prevent many of these eye diseases later in life. This is just one way that Saratoga Retina is working to promote eye health.

I have made my home in beautiful Saratoga Springs, New York seeing patients from Glens Falls, Saratoga, Albany and the surrounding area. I continue to strive to improve the patient's experience and am developing my own Surgery Centers in Saratoga Springs, New York, in Amman, Jordan and in Dubai, United Arab Emirates. These surgery centers will be dedicated to the advancement of eye surgery providing patients with the absolute best possible experience, treatment options and outcomes.

Introduction:

First and foremost, I am sorry that you have to read this book, but I am glad that you are here. I have heard countless times how frightening it is to lose your vision and how patients have laid awake at night worrying about what is going to happen. Like so many things, we take our eyesight for granted until it is lost. Since 1994, I have been treating patients with retinal diseases. What I have seen first hand is the importance of early detection and treatment.

Our goal at Saratoga Retina is to help you find the answers and treatment plan for your symptoms. But more importantly, we want to help you get your quality of life back so you can continue to do all the activities you so enjoy. We will help you understand the causes of your eye problems and will help guide you to healthy eye care.

As the years go by, I realized that what patients really want is a treatment plan they can understand and answers to their questions in a way they understand. And what patients really need is someone to guide them through the treatment process and provide the comfort they need. That is where Saratoga Retina comes in. I know you will love my staff as much as I do. They are incredibly caring and dedicated to your comfort and care.

Chapter 1

You've been told you need a Retina Specialist: Three Important Points To Get You Started

First: don't worry!

A retina specialist is a medical doctor who has specialized in ophthalmology and is a highly trained subspecialist in diseases and surgery of the vitreous body of the eye and the retina. This subspecialty is sometimes known as vitreoretinal medicine. These special skills allow us to diagnose and treat specific parts of the highly complex human visual system. Diagnosis of retina and vitreous diseases may require highly technical equipment and testing as well as thorough examination.

Retina specialists must complete medical school and specialized training as an ophthalmologist, and then pursue additional vitreoretinal training. The full breadth of training for a retina specialist includes:

- Undergraduate College: 4 years

- Medical School - 4 years

- Internship - 1 year

- Ophthalmology Residency - 3 years

- Retina-Vitreous Fellowship - 2 years

The medical treatments and surgical procedures used by retina specialists are extremely exacting and delicate. Most of the surgeries require a microscope and are therefore microsurgical procedures. Retinal specialists work on extremely delicate tissues in an incredibly small space. The laser is a vital part of the medical tools available to us and there are many office and hospital procedures in which we will use a laser.

We treat a variety of conditions and diseases, ranging from age-related macular degeneration to retinal detachment and cancers of the eye, working with both adults and children. As a retina specialist, we may also treat a patient who has experienced severe eye trauma and may be consulted in the case of patients dealing with hereditary diseases of the eye.

Some of the surgeries retina specialists perform are:

- Retinal Detachment Surgery

- Diabetic Vitrectomy

- Macular Pucker Vitrectomy

- Macular Hole Vitrectomy

- Repair of Ruptured Globe

<u>Second</u>: don't be intimidated.

Your health and eyesight is too important! Doctors are people too and understand what you are going through. It's perfectly normal to be frightened and overwhelmed. We are here to guide you through your treatment options. We want to know what is on your mind and any concerns you may have.

It is my goal to provide the very best and most up to date care I can in an environment that brings you comfort and ease. I want you to feel empowered in your own health and will take the time to ensure you understand your treatment plan.

I am honored that my staff tells all our patients, "Not to worry, this is where I would send my Mom or Dad!" That is my goal to treat you like family and provide service in a timely manner. We don't overbook our patients and work very hard every day to stay on schedule for your appointment. We respect your time!

Third: write down your questions and don't be afraid to ask.

You need to also ask yourself, "What are my concerns?" "What am I worried about?" Be careful of the medical advice you get from family and friends. The vision problem your neighbor's second cousin had may not need the same treatment plan you do.

We know that you may have the same questions multiple times. It is important to us that you feel comfortable in our office and surgery center; so don't be afraid to write down what you are thinking so that when you get to your appointment you don't forget to ask. Many times my staff will even answer your questions before you even ask them!

Chapter 2

Choosing The Right Retina Specialist: The Bottom Line Is You Must Find A Specialist You Like And Trust

Now you must decide whom to choose. This decision alone can be daunting as we have to put so much faith in our Doctor's hands. And in this case, your vision depends on it. Here are three basic steps to follow to help you decide which Retina Specialist is right for you.

Step 1: Get the name of the Retina Specialist that your Ophthalmologist, Optometrist, or Primary Care Physician recommends. This is going to be someone that they trust and have seen great results with. When someone continues to refer to the same specialist, you know that the patients are happy and well taken care of.

Step 2: Do some research and gather the names of potential doctors. Research simply means to look on the Internet, check out the Yellow Pages and talk to family, friends and co-workers.

The Internet contains a library of information right at your fingertips and will provide you with a world of information. For example, go online to my website www.SaratogaRetina.com and you will find an example of what I'm talking about. On my website, I provide all kinds of free information about your vision that is designed to answer your questions. My goal is to educate.

Ask yourself some questions:

Is the Retina Specialist Board Certified? It is important that they pass the rigorous examinations to continue to meet the state and federal requirements to practice medicine.

Are they at the top of their field and educate others by teaching, speaking and writing? These activities show that they are key opinion leaders and continue their education to stay on the cutting edge and pass that knowledge on to others in their field.

You want to put your care in the hands of a doctor that cares for your ailment day in and day out, loves what they do and wants to continue their education well after they get out of school.

Step 3: Call the office.

The first impression of the doctor can be seen through his staff. Are you treated with respect and dignity? Many of your questions, concerns and follow up may be directed to staff members and you must be comfortable and confident in their presence as well. Would the staff send their family members to see this physician? The staff knows the doctor the best and wouldn't send a loved one to someone they didn't trust!

Chapter 3

Macular Degeneration, Diabetic Retinopathy and Retinal Detachment:

Three common diseases of the eye and what it means for you

Let's first look at what a healthy eye consists of:

A healthy retina is necessary for good vision. The eye is composed of light-sensitive cells connected with nerve fibers that allow light entering the eye to be converted to nerve impulses that reach the brain. The amount of light entering is controlled by the iris, which is then passed to the retina.

The retina is a light-sensitive area in the back of the eye, and it includes the macula, which is made up of light-sensitive cells that give us our ability to have sharp, detailed vision. In a healthy eye, images are focused onto the retina and then converted into electrical signals that are sent to the brain by the optic nerve for processing.

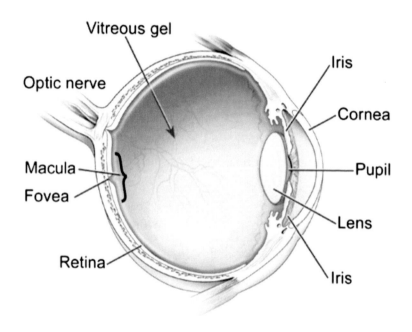

The vitreous body of the eye is a clear gel, which fills the space between the retina and the lens. The retina, the macula and the vitreous body can all be subject to diseases and conditions that can lead to blindness or vision interruption and may require the attention of a retina specialist.

To examine the retina, your eyes will be dilated during a comprehensive examination. To dilate or widen your eyes, drops are placed in them. I will then use a special magnifying lens to examine your retina. The dilation will reverse after several hours.

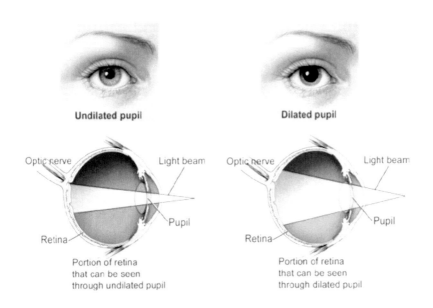

Undilated pupil

Dilated pupil

Optic nerve   Light beam

Optic nerve   Light beam

Pupil

Pupil

Retina

Retina

Portion of retina
that can be seen
through undilated pupil

Portion of retina
that can be seen
through dilated pupil

Age-related Macular Degeneration

Age-related Macular Degeneration (AMD) is the leading cause of blindness and loss of central vision among adults over the age of 65. AMD is a chronic disease that affects the retina – the part of the eye that allows you to see fine detail -- blurring your central vision. It can have devastating impact on your ability to read, drive, or engage in other activities of daily life. An estimated 15 million North Americans alone have AMD.

AMD view

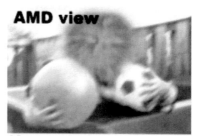

Normal view

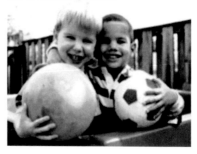

There are two forms of AMD, known as "dry" and "wet":

• **Dry AMD** - Characterized by small yellow particles and pigment changes in the macula caused by cells breaking down. Over time, the deposits may grow together and harden, thereby interfering with central vision.

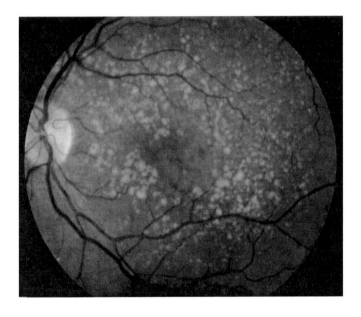

Dry AMD

- **Wet AMD** - Occurs when abnormal blood vessels behind the retina start to grow under the macula. These blood vessels often leak blood and fluid. Wet AMD is the more advanced form of the disease and loss of vision occurs quickly.

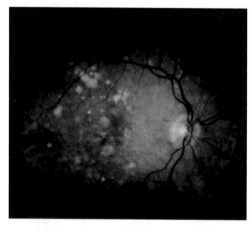

Early Stage Wet AMD

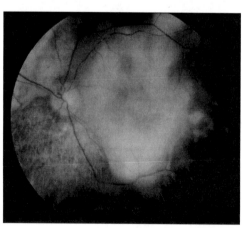

End Stage Wet AMD

Most patients have what is called the "dry" form, in which the yellow deposits, called drusen, are present in the macula. In advanced stages, tissue death may lead to blind spots and loss of central vision. About 10 percent of people with AMD develop the "wet" form of the disease in which abnormal blood vessels grow.

Symptoms

The earliest signs of macular degeneration in the retina can be detected before you have any vision loss. This detection is facilitated by an eye exam in which eye drops are given to dilate the pupil of the eye.

Patients with macular degeneration are usually older than 55 years old, have signs of macular degeneration in both of their eyes and may have experienced some slow, insidious vision loss. Most have dry macular degeneration. Perhaps 85 – 90% of macular degeneration is of the "dry" variety.

Dry AMD usually occurs slowly, over time. The patient may notice a need for brighter light when reading. Other symptoms may include difficulty adapting to low light levels, increased blurriness of printed words, decrease in brightness of colors, or a blurred spot in the center of the field of vision. A dark blank or black spot in the middle of your vision can also be a sign of macular degeneration. This spot starts out small, grows over time and could eventually lead to legal blindness in your central vision but does not affect your peripheral or side vision. So you never become totally blind.

In contrast, visual changes in wet AMD occur more rapidly, resulting in an abrupt decline in central vision. Patients may experience visual distortions, such as straight lines appearing wavy, or objects appearing larger or smaller than they are. As in dry AMD, patients may also notice a well-defined blind spot in the center of vision.

You should also keep an eye out for early symptoms of macular degeneration. Here are some things to look for:

Watch for straight lines that appear broken, crooked, wavy, bent or distorted in your vision. One way to test your eye sight is to use an **Amsler Grid.**

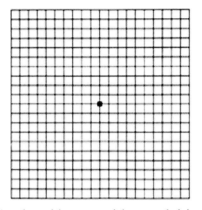

Amsler grid as seen with normal vision

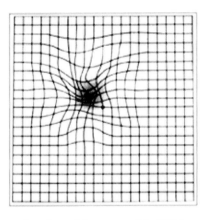

Amsler grid as seen with AMD

If the lines in the grid appear anything but straight and unbroken, you might be experiencing a typical symptom of macular degeneration.

However, this test is hardly sufficient to rule out the possibility that one has developed macular degeneration. Many people with macular degeneration may see no abnormalities on an Amsler grid, so don't use this as a substitute for regular good dilated eye examinations of the retina.

Pay close attention to a decline in your central vision, both close-up and distant. People use central vision when they drive, read, look at faces or view pictures. Your central vision allows you to see details, colors and shapes more clearly.

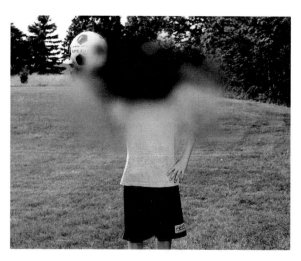

AMD causes patchy vision that often interferes with visual efficiency

Regular dilated eye exams with an ophthalmologist are important, especially when you're at higher risk for macular degeneration. If you are over the age of 50, an exam every one to two years is a good idea in order to look for signs of macular degeneration before any vision loss has occurred.

Causes

AMD is caused by the destruction of light-sensitive cells in the macula. The macula is the central portion of the retina in the back of the eye. The light-sensitive cells of the macula give us our ability to have sharp, detailed vision.

In a healthy eye, images are focused onto the retina and then converted into electrical signals that are sent to the brain for processing. During normal aging, yellowish deposits, called drusen, form under the retina. It is possible to have drusen with no accompanying loss of vision.

But as drusen increase in size and number, they can interfere with proper functioning of the retina, damaging or killing the light-sensitive cells of the macula. This is how dry AMD occurs.

The wet form of AMD occurs when blood vessels behind the retina begin to grow in an abnormal way. These newly formed blood vessels can then leak blood and fluid, causing the macula to swell. Again, the macula's light-sensitive cells are damaged or killed.

Risk factors

The primary risk factor for AMD is age. The older you are, the greater your risk for macular degeneration. Also, people with a family history of the disease are at higher risk for macular degeneration, as are women, and people of European descent.

Diagnostic tests

One way to check for AMD is to look at an Amsler Grid as shown earlier in this chapter. Cover one eye and stare at the black dot in the center. If the straight lines appear wavy or are missing you may have AMD.

A fluorescein angiogram is usually performed to demonstrate

the presence of neovascularization. If present, therapy may be instituted soon, to prevent further vision loss. The earlier the diagnosis is made, the better.

Fluorescein Angiography

Angiography is a diagnostic procedure in which a rapid sequence of photographs is taken to document the blood circulation of the retina. In this test, illuminated dye is injected into the body through your veins, usually in the arm, forearm or hand. As your blood flows, the dye gradually appears in the retina.

Since the fluorescein dye is a very bright yellow, the skin may appear jaundiced for a few hours and then the yellow color disappears. The dye is excreted through the kidneys causing the urine to be a bright yellow for 24-36 hours. The coloration of this dye is considered to be a normal result of the after effects.

I will photograph the retina and evaluate its appearance with the help of the illuminated dye. This analysis helps determine if the disease is present and how far it has progressed.

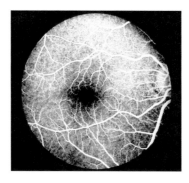

Normal eye as seen in fluorescein angiography

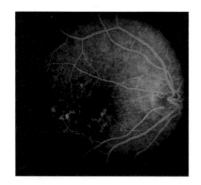 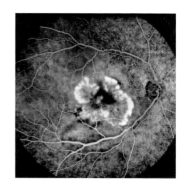

Dry AMD   Wet AMD

as seen in fluorescein angiography

Optical Coherence Tomography (OCT)

This latest generation of imaging technology makes quicker and more accurate diagnoses possible. Instead of using acoustic waves as in ultrasound, OCT uses light to take cross section images of the retina and is 15 times more sensitive than conventional ultrasound.

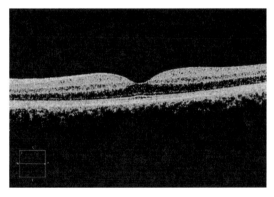

Normal eye seen with OCT scan

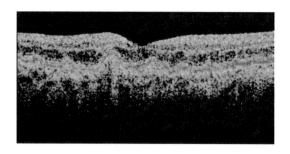

Dry AMD seen with OCT scan

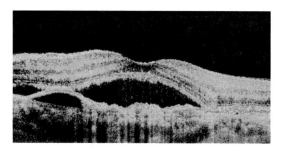

Wet AMD seen with OCT scan

B-Scan Ultrasound

B-Scan ultrasound is most useful when direct visualization of intraocular structures is difficult or impossible. Situations that prevent normal examination include lid problems, severe edema, corneal opacities, dense cataracts or hemorrhage. In such cases, diagnostic B-scan ultrasound can give valuable information on the status of the vitreous and retina.

Treatment and drugs

There is no known cure for AMD. However, through early detection and proper treatment AMD patients can protect their vision from further deterioration. More advanced stages can often now be treated, as well.

Currently, no medical treatments exist for dry AMD, but I may suggest strategies to slow its progression – taking vitamin or mineral supplements, for example.

It is extremely important to continue to get regular eye examinations, especially if you have been diagnosed with dry AMD. If you experience new symptoms, or your vision suddenly deteriorates, you should see a retina specialist right away.

A variety of medical treatments are now available for wet AMD. None of them are considered a cure, but they can help stop further vision loss. Treatment options include laser surgery, photodynamic therapy, or injections aimed at destroying abnormal blood vessels or preventing them from leaking. Most often, I treat "wet" macular degeneration with anti-VEGF intraocular injections.

Prevention

Can AMD be prevented? Like most things in life, there is no easy answer.

Age and genetics are both linked to the likelihood of being diagnosed with AMD. Older people, those from a family with a history of the disease and those of European descent are at higher risk for macular degeneration. Unfortunately, there is nothing we can do about these factors.

However, some lifestyle factors are also known to increase your risk for AMD. If you alter these factors, you may decrease the chance of getting macular degeneration. The most important modifiable risk factor is cigarette smoking. Obesity, hypertension (high blood pressure), excessive sun exposure and a diet deficient in fruits and vegetables also might increase your risk.

Eliminating these factors, of course, not only may reduce your risk for macular degeneration, but for many other things as well, including cancer and cardiovascular disease.

While no cure exists for AMD yet, treatments can slow its progression if it is detected early.

Most important of all keep this in mind: You can still have a good quality of life, even with a diagnosis of macular degeneration. Even though AMD makes it harder to see, it only rarely leads to complete blindness. While it can be a difficult condition, it is usually not as devastating to people as they fear when initially diagnosed.

Most patients are able to keep some of their vision, and they learn to adapt, finding ways to use their remaining vision to its fullest capacity. Millions of Americans are living healthy and independent lives, despite having AMD.

Diabetic Retinopathy

One of the most frequent causes of vision impairment in the United States and throughout the rest of the world is diabetic retinopathy. Diabetic retinopathy is a complication of diabetes that causes damage to the blood vessels of the retina – the light-sensitive tissue that lines the back part of the eye, allowing you to see fine detail. Diabetic retinopathy occurs in more than half of the people who develop diabetes. The longer you have diabetes and the less controlled your blood sugar is, the more likely the possibility that you will develop diabetic retinopathy.

There are generally two causes of vision loss from diabetic retinopathy – diabetic macular edema and proliferative diabetic retinopathy.

- **Diabetic macular edema**. Diabetic macular edema is the term used for swelling in the central part of the retina. The macula, or center part, of the retina is used for sharp, straight-ahead vision. It is nourished by blood vessels that become affected by diabetes. The blood vessels are weakened by diabetes and may become leaky. This causes the retina to become thickened or swollen. It is this swelling of the central part of the retina that can lead to decreased vision.

- **Proliferative diabetic retinopathy**. Diabetes can cause damage to the small blood vessels in the retina, resulting in poor circulation to the retina. Vision may be lost because some of the retina tissue may die as a result of this inadequate blood supply. Unlike skin tissue, which might grow back if it is lost, retina tissue is like brain tissue and does not grow back once it is lost. Furthermore, the poor circulation may lead to the development of growth factors that can cause new blood vessels and scar tissue to grow on the surface of the retina.

This stage of diabetic retinopathy is called proliferative diabetic retinopathy (PDR). It is referred to as "proliferative" because at this stage of the disease, new, abnormal blood vessels and scar tissue begin to grow on the surface of the retina. The vessels bleed into the middle cavity of the eye, causing vision loss because light cannot reach the retina. In addition, the scar tissue formation can pull on the retina and cause vision loss by detaching the retina from the back of the eye. Occasionally, these blood vessels and scar tissue may grow in the front of the eye, where fluid normally exits. When the fluid cannot escape, pressure can build in the eye, creating a rare type of glaucoma (neovascular glaucoma) that can damage the vision even further and cause the eye to become painful.

Symptoms

It is possible to have diabetic retinopathy for a long time without noticing symptoms. Often, diabetic retinopathy will cause changes unnoticeable to a patient until substantial damage already has occurred.

Diabetic retinopathy usually affects both eyes. Symptoms may include blurred or double vision, difficulty reading, or the appearance of spots – known as "floaters" – in your vision. You also may notice a shadow across your field of vision, pain or pressure in your eyes, or difficulty with color perception. Some patients may experience a partial or total loss of vision.

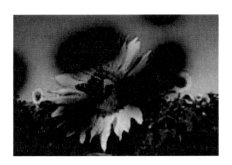

Causes

The primary cause of diabetic retinopathy is diabetes – a condition in which the levels of glucose (sugar) in your blood are too high. Elevated sugar levels from diabetes can damage the small blood vessels that nourish the retina, and may in some cases block them completely. As a result, the blood supply to the retina from these damaged blood vessels is cut off, and vision is affected.

As mentioned above, in response to the lack of blood supply

the eye may create growth factors that cause leakage of blood vessels that result in swelling of the retina (diabetic macular edema) or growth of new blood vessels and scar tissue (proliferative diabetic retinopathy). These new blood vessels can bleed into the middle cavity of the eye, and the scar tissue can pull on the retina -- sometimes, leading to vision loss if the retina detaches from the back wall of the eye.

Risk factors

Anyone who has diabetes is at risk of developing diabetic retinopathy. There are, however, additional factors that can increase your risk.

One of the most important factors is the duration of your diabetes. The longer you have had it, the greater your risk of developing diabetic retinopathy. Another key factor is how well you have controlled your blood sugar level over time. Another factor that can influence the control of your blood sugar level and the subsequent development of diabetic retinopathy is high blood pressure. It also is possible that cholesterol levels can have an effect on this process, and pregnancy in someone with diabetes can result in changes in the retina as well.

Diagnostic tests

The best way to diagnose diabetic retinopathy is with a dilated eye exam. During the exam, you will receive drops in your eyes to make your pupils dilate (open widely) to allow a better view of the inside of your eye, especially the retina tissue.

During the exam, I will look for swelling in the retina (diabetic macular edema), abnormal blood vessels that may predict an increased risk of developing new blood vessels, and the actual presence of new blood vessels or scar tissue on the surface of the retina (proliferative diabetic retinopathy).

Three other diagnostic tools are also used to detect and manage diabetic retinopathy:

• **Fundus photography.** I may take photographs of the back of the eye to facilitate detection of diabetic retinopathy as well as to document the retinopathy to make it easier to determine if the condition is worsening at a subsequent visit.

• **Fluorescein angiography**. To supplement the eye exam, I may conduct a retinal photography test called fluorescein angiography. After dilating your pupils, a dye will be injected into your arm that will circulate through your eyes. It is like a food coloring however, it does not affect the kidneys, and is unlike the dye that is used with MRIs or CAT scans. As the dye circulates, pictures are taken of the retina, allowing me to accurately detect blood vessels that are closed, damaged, or leaking fluid. The pictures are black and white to facilitate the detection of these changes, but the process is not the same as having an x-ray.

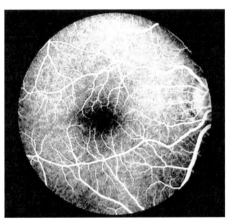

Normal eye under Fluorescein Angiography

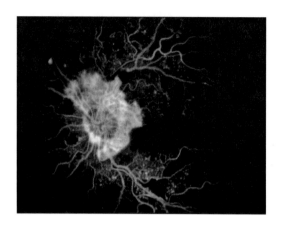

Diabetic Retinopathy under Fluorescein Angiography

Optical coherence tomography (OCT): I may suggest an optical coherence tomography (OCT) exam. This test provides cross-sectional images of the retina that show its thickness, helping determine whether fluid has leaked into retinal tissue. This latest generation of imaging technology (15 times more sensitive than conventional ultrasound) makes quicker and more accurate diagnoses possible. Instead of using acoustic waves as in ultrasound, OCT uses light to take cross section images of the retina.

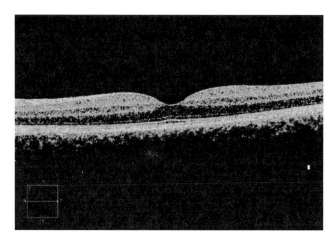

Normal eye seen with OCT scan

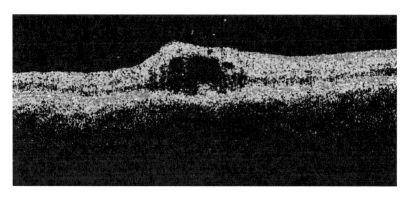

Diabetic Retinopathy seen with OCT scan

B-Scan Ultrasound

B-Scan ultrasound is most useful when direct visualization of intraocular structures is difficult or impossible. Situations that prevent normal examination include lid problems, severe edema, corneal opacities, dense cataracts or hemorrhage. In such cases, diagnostic B-scan ultrasound can give valuable information on the status of the vitreous and retina.

Treatment and drugs

There now are many treatments for diabetic retinopathy, including lasers to the retina or miniscule injections of medications into the middle cavity of the eye. These procedures can be done in my office to prevent, treat, or reverse damage from diabetes in the retina.

Researchers have shown that eye injections, often but not always in combination with laser treatment, result in better vision than laser treatment alone for diabetes-associated swelling of the retina—the condition known as diabetic macular edema.

The key to these treatments is the blocking by eye injections of a chemical signal in the body that stimulates blood vessel growth, known as vascular endothelial growth factor (VEGF).

Repeated doses of anti-VEGF medications may be needed to prevent blood vessels from leaking fluid and causing damage to the eye.

I commonly treat patients with "focal" laser photocoagulation for diabetic macular edema. This occurs in most patients. The laser has been a great tool for preventing additional leakage, thereby preserving visual acuity. At times, there are situations that are not amenable to treatment with laser and we may discuss the possibility of intravitreal (aka intraocular) injections of steroids or anti-VEGF medicines.

Patients who have developed the proliferative phase of diabetic retinopathy may require PRP, or pan-retinal photocoagulation. The laser is used in this instance to treat the peripheral retina. Enough PRP is treated to reverse the neovascular tissue growing along the surface of the retina. Once the proliferative phase of the diabetic retinopathy is arrested, the chance of blindness is dramatically reduced.

With proper examinations, the earliest signs of diabetic

retinopathy in the retina can be detected before you have any vision loss.

Regular dilated eye exams with a retina specialist are important, especially when you're at higher risk for diabetic retinopathy or diabetes. Over the age of 50, an exam every year is a good idea to look for signs of diabetes or diabetic retinopathy before any vision loss has occurred.

Even if not all vision loss from diabetic retinopathy can be prevented or treated at this time, patients usually are able to find ways to live with diminished vision.

Prevention

Patients with diabetes frequently ask, "Is there anything I can do to keep from getting diabetic retinopathy or to prevent or treat vision loss once it occurs from diabetic retinopathy?"

The answer is a resounding yes.

First, the better your control of diabetes – controlling your blood sugar levels through diet, exercise and medications, the less likely you will develop diabetic retinopathy or have worsening of any pre-existing retinopathy. One of the best ways to monitor your blood sugar levels is by having your health care provider who manages your diabetes evaluate your hemoglobin A1C, which is measured through a blood test obtained in the office. This will help you keep your blood sugar levels in a target range.

Second, control of your blood pressure and possibly your lipid levels can affect the impact of diabetes on your retina.

Finally, avoid delayed diagnosis and treatment. Eye exams are extremely important. Getting a dilated eye exam won't prevent retinopathy, but it certainly can reduce your risk of more severe complications from the disease, should it develop. By detecting it early, you can get treatment that will help prevent vision loss and slow the disease's progression. You should schedule regular eye exams, and see a retina specialist if you are told that you have diabetic retinopathy.

It has been my experience that most patients with diabetic

retinopathy actually do well over their lifetime, that is, most patients are able to retain good, useful vision. The patients that have had the most difficulty with permanent loss of vision, including blindness are those that wait way too long to see an eye doctor. Prevention with this disease is paramount.

If you have been diagnosed with diabetes, please request a copy of my book, "Diabetes And Your Eye: 7 Steps To Prevention & Control of Diabetic Eye Conditions" where I go into more detail on how to prevent and manage diabetic eye diseases. You can request a copy here http://www.SaratogaRetina.com

Retinal Detachment

Retinal detachments can be pretty frightening. Often, I don't get to see a patient soon enough as most hope the symptoms will "just go away." Basically, the earlier I can diagnose and manage a retinal detachment, the better chance of doing well. If not treated promptly a retinal detachment can result in permanent vision loss. A detachment occurs when the retina is lifted or pulled from its normal position in the eye. It may begin with a small tear or break that leads to a full detachment. It is extremely important to recognize that a retinal detachment is a medical emergency and should be treated as one.

Signs of a detachment or tear include a sudden or gradual increase in floaters or specks that float in your field of vision. It may also begin with a curtain over the field of vision.

There are three different types of retinal detachment:

Rhegmatogenous [reg-ma-TAH-jenous] - A tear or break in the retina allows fluid to get under the retina and separate it from the retinal pigment epithelium (RPE), the pigmented cell layer that nourishes the retina. These types of retinal detachments are the most common.

Tractional - In this type of detachment, scar tissue on the retina's surface contracts and causes the retina to separate from the RPE. This type of detachment is less common.

Exudative - In this type, fluid leaks into the area underneath the retina, but there are no tears or breaks in the retina. Frequently caused by retinal diseases, including inflammatory disorders and injury/trauma to the eye.

Causes and Risk Factors

A detached retina usually stems from a retinal tear or retinal hole. Occasionally there is a history of trauma. Retinal detachments usually happen in normal, healthy individuals. Surgery is required in most cases and is about 90-95% successful in reattaching the retina. Visual return is dependent upon age, length of detachment and involvement of the macula.

A retinal detachment can occur at any age, but it is more common in people over age 40. It affects men more than women, and Whites more than African Americans.

A retinal detachment is also more likely to occur in people who:

• Are extremely nearsighted
• Have had a retinal detachment in the other eye
• Have a family history of retinal detachment
• Have had cataract surgery
• Have other eye diseases or disorders, such as retinoschisis, uveitis, degenerative myopia, or lattice degeneration
• Have had an eye injury

Symptoms and Detection

Symptoms include a sudden or gradual increase in either the number of floaters, which are little "cobwebs" or specks that float about in your field of vision, and/or light flashes in the eye. Another symptom is the appearance of a curtain over the field of vision. **A retinal detachment is a medical emergency.** Anyone experiencing the symptoms of a retinal detachment should see an eye care professional immediately.

Treatment

The natural course of a retinal detachment is blindness. On rare occasion, with time, there may be loss of the eye. So there really isn't much choice, but to operate in an attempt to repair the detached retina. Surgery for a retinal detachment is usually urgent. The timing and urgency of surgery depends upon the macula. If the macula is attached (the best situation), surgery may be scheduled before the macula becomes detached. If the macula is already detached (central vision is now reduced or absent), the timing is less imperative. This sounds a bit counter-intuitive I know.

Small holes and tears are treated with laser surgery or a freeze treatment called cryopexy. During laser surgery tiny burns are made around the hole to "weld" the retina back into place. Cryopexy freezes the area around the hole and helps reattach the retina.

Retinal detachments are treated with surgery involving a vitrectomy or a scleral buckle, or both.

During a scleral buckle, a tiny synthetic band is attached to the outside of the eyeball to gently push the wall of the eye against the detached retina. If necessary, a vitrectomy may also be performed.

During a vitrectomy, the doctor makes tiny incisions in the sclera (white of the eye). Next, a small instrument is placed into the eye to remove the vitreous, a gel-like substance that fills the center of the eye and helps the eye maintain a round shape. Gas is often injected to into the eye to replace the vitreous and reattach the retina; the gas pushes the retina back against the wall of the eye. During the healing process, the eye makes fluid that gradually replaces the gas and fills the eye.

I will discuss having a vitrectomy in more detail in Chapter 6.

With modern therapy, over 90 percent of those with a retinal detachment can be successfully treated, although sometimes a second or third surgery is needed. However, the visual outcome is not always predictable. The final visual result may not be known for up to several months following surgery. Even under the best of circumstances, and even after multiple attempts at repair, treatment sometimes fails and vision may eventually be lost. Visual results are best if the retinal detachment is repaired before the macula (the center region of the retina responsible for fine, detailed vision) detaches. That is why it is important to contact an eye care professional immediately if you see a sudden or gradual increase in the number of floaters and/or light flashes, or a dark curtain over the field of vision.

Chapter 4

7 Questions Your Retina Specialist Will Ask You At Your First Appointment

Getting regular eye exams is very important to your health. Seeing a retina specialist is very similar to other medical doctor appointments. However, this appointment can be more frightening because your vision is involved and blindness is something we never expected to think about.

In order to prepare for your first visit, here are 7 questions you should be ready to answer.

1. Who referred you to our practice?

Since we are a specialist office we do not generally see patients unless they have a retina associated problem. So we are interested in knowing that you have been seen by another doctor and that they recommended you be seen by a specialist. We are also interested in ensuring we provide the best possible follow-up information and updates to the physician that sent you to us.

2. Have you been diagnosed with Macular Degeneration?

If you were not referred by your physician, but have been previously diagnosed with macular degeneration you are a good candidate for our practice.

3. Have you been diagnosed with diabetes?

Diabetes can greatly affect your vision and the best prevention is getting regular eye exams from your retina specialist and controlling your blood sugar. It is important that we begin seeing you as soon as possible after your diagnosis.

4. What symptoms are you experiencing?

As we grow older, definite changes occur in our vision. These vision changes can sometimes limit activities of daily life, such as reading, driving and hobbies. It is important for us to know all the symptoms you are experiencing and how they are affecting you.

5. What other conditions do you manage?

As your retina specialist, it is important for us to know what other conditions you are currently being treated for as that can have an impact not only on what is causing your vision loss but also on how we treat it.

6. What medications are you currently taking?

You know the drill...we always need to know what medications you are on so that we can avoid any contraindications. In addition, some medications can cause vision impairment and for this reason we are acutely interested in what you are taking!

7. What concerns do you have?

You are the most important member of your health care team and responsible for executing and following your doctors' instructions.

After all, you are the one who is affected by vision loss and manages it every day. Only you know how you feel and what you're willing and able to do. This is very important and will lead me right into the next chapter.

Chapter 5

The Fifteen Critical Questions You Should Ask Your Retina Specialist

As I stated in Chapter 1, don't worry, don't be intimidated and write your questions down! I can't stress this enough. As much as I want you to relax before your appointments with me I know you will be nervous or frightened. I get that. Vision loss is scary and can affect your daily routine.

So in order for you to get the most out of your appointment, you need to be prepared to ask questions. The only way to remember what you wanted to ask is to write it down! We get many great questions from our patients. Here are the most frequently asked questions that you may want to ask at your appointment as well.

1. **How long will my appointment take?**

   We respect you time and strive to take you back for your appointment within 15 minutes of your scheduled time. You should expect your appointment to last 1 1/2 hours.

2. **Will I need a driver or can I drive myself?**

   You will need to come to your appointment with someone else to drive you home. Even though you have probably had a dilated eye exam before, this will be different and as my staff will tell you, this is a "super dilated" exam that can take hours to wear off.

3. **How soon will I be seen?**

   Based on what you are being seen for will determine how urgent the appointment is. Generally, we will book your appointment within 2 weeks, but some conditions need to be seen within 48 hours or the most acute conditions need a same day appointment.

4. **Will I have surgery when I'm there in the office?**

Usually not, some procedures are done right in the office, but your first appointment will be a thorough eye exam to determine an accurate diagnosis and map out your treatment plan.

5. **Do I need to bring anything to the appointment?**

Your referring physician will send the needed information to our office and a thorough exam will be done at your appointment. We do need you to know what medications you are on and general questions regarding your overall health.

6. **Will it hurt?**

I'm asked this a lot. Generally speaking, no you won't feel any of the procedures and your exams are painless. We use anesthetic drops when necessary. Even during injections, most people say that they didn't even know when the injection was happening.

7. Will my vision get better?

This is a great question and one that is on everyone's mind and should be asked. You may also be thinking "Will I go blind?" Not all vision can be restored and success can sometimes be stopping vision loss from getting worse.

8. When can I go back to work?

This answer will vary based on the procedure.

9. How long will my treatments take?

This answer will vary on the condition you have been diagnosed with, but we will go through your treatment plan with you in detail at your appointment.

10. What eye drops do I need to take?

No eye drops are necessary to take prior to your initial exam. If you are prescribed eye drops during your appointment, I will give you a prescription during your exam.

11.   How do I take my eye drops?

The need for drops is dependent on the procedure. If you do require drops here is an effective way to put drops in your eye.

1. Tilt you head back
2. Create a pocket by pulling down on your lower lid
3. Put one drop of the medication in the lower lid pocket
4. Gently close BOTH eyes, Do not squeeze or blink
5. Count to 30, allowing the medication to be absorbed
6. If more than one medication has been prescribed, wait at least 5 minutes and follow steps 1-5.

12.   Can you fill out my Motor Vehicle form?

We generally do not fill out the forms for you. Your general eye doctor is responsible for that.

13.   Can I shower after my laser or injection procedure?

We recommend no water or soap 24 hours after your procedure.

14. When can I go back to the gym after having a laser or injection procedure?

This depends on your condition so be sure to ask Dr. Jay.

15. Is there anything special I should do after my appointment?

Your dilation will take several hours to wear off, so be sure to have sunglasses available to shield your eyes from bright light. If you are having a procedure, you will receive specific instructions at that time.

Chapter 6

I've Been Scheduled For Surgery - What Should I Expect?

The vitreous is normally a clear, jelly-like fluid that fills the inside of the eye. Various disease states that we have discussed can cause the vitreous to cloud, fill with blood or even harden so that light entering the eye will be misdirected and not reach the retina properly.

When this occurs, a vitrectomy may be required. A vitrectomy is a surgical procedure that removes the vitreous in the central cavity of the eye so that vision can be corrected. It is beneficial in many disease states including diabetic retinopathy, retinal detachments, macular holes, macular puckers and vitreous hemorrhage.

The vitrectomy procedure is usually performed as an outpatient procedure in a hospital or surgery center setting. Local anesthesia is common and general anesthesia may rarely be used. The eye will be held open using a special speculum and the eye that is not being operated on will be covered.

I begin the procedure by making a small (less than 1mm) opening in the side of the eye and inserting an infusion line to maintain constant eye pressure. Next a microscopic cutting device is inserted which will cut and aspirate (suck out) the vitreous fluid.

A microscopic light source is also inserted to illuminate the inside of the eye through the procedure. Additional instruments may also be used to perform maneuvers such as cauterizing blood vessel leaks or removing scar tissue.

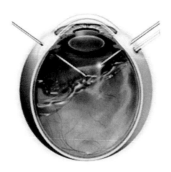

Vitrectomy Illustration

I will be looking through a microscope while performing the procedure and may also use special lenses to help see the anatomy of the eye. After the vitreous is removed, I will refill the eye with a special saline solution that closely resembles the natural vitreous fluid in your eye.

Normal vitrectomy healing time is between 4 to 6 weeks. Normal restoration of vision can take several weeks. Physical activity will be restricted during this time to prevent any complications.

Postoperative Instructions:

Since vitrectomy is often performed along with other procedures, postoperative instruction may vary and I will give you specific instructions at the time of surgery. However, some general guidelines:

1. Begin using any anti-inflammatory and antibiotic drops as prescribed immediately after your eye patch has been removed. (You will receive all necessary drops at your appointment the day after surgery.)

2. Wear the plastic shield when sleeping for the first 7 days following surgery.

3. Avoid bending, stooping, lifting objects over 15 pounds, or any strenuous activity for one week.

4. Take Tylenol Extra Strength or gently apply ice compresses to the eye to relieve mild discomfort.

5. Follow any special instructions given for head positioning (this is not necessary in all cases).

Frequently Asked Questions Regarding Your Surgery:

How long does the surgery take?

Your surgery will generally take between 30-45 minutes.

Will I feel the surgery?

You will have anesthesia during the surgery and only minimal discomfort after the surgery.

What type of anesthesia will I have?

For most surgeries, our patients have Monitored Anesthesia Care (MAC) anesthesia. This is an IV anesthesia where you will be awake and relaxed. You will be able to hear people talking in the operating room. You will be able to speak, but you shouldn't because when your lips move your eyes move! If you have had a colonoscopy, this is the same type of anesthesia.

Do I need to pick up any medication prior to surgery?

No, you will receive a post-operative kit at your first visit, the day after surgery with everything you need. There is no need to go to the pharmacy, simply go home and rest.

Will I wear an eye patch?

Yes, you will wake up wearing an eye patch and continuing wearing it for the first night after the surgery.

Will I have to be in a certain position after surgery?

Not all surgeries require special positioning. Some do and you will have 7-10 days of special positioning as the retina reattaches.

Will I need eye drops after surgery?

Yes, you will use eye drops for a few weeks following your surgery.

How long will I stay in the hospital after surgery?

All of the surgeries are outpatient procedures. Patients do not usually need to stay in the hospital overnight following surgery. We will remove the eye patch and examine your eye the morning after surgery in our office.

Will I have to return to Saratoga Retina for follow-up appointments?

Yes, I will need to monitor your eye as it heals. Many of your appointments will require special testing that will give me valuable information regarding your vision. Most patients return for four visits during the first six months following surgery.

Do I need a driver?

You will need someone to drive you to and from the surgery center and to and from your appointment in my office the next day.

How many surgeries has Dr. Jay has performed?

Dr. Jay worldwide has performed more than three thousand retinal surgeries. He has also trained and supervised other physicians on thousands more.

If I have received photodynamic therapy (PDT) -- or Avastin, Lucentis, or other medicines to stop the blood vessels - am I still a candidate for surgery?

Yes, you can still be a candidate. Some patients who still have poor vision after other treatments have recovered central vision after surgery.

Chapter 7

I've Been Scheduled For Injections or Laser Treatment -
What Should I Expect?

Laser treatment typically requires no overnight hospital stay, so you will be treated on an outpatient basis in my office.

Make sure you have someone drive you to and from the office on the day you have the procedure. Also, you'll need to wear sunglasses afterward because your eyes will be temporarily dilated and light sensitive.

Before the procedure, you will receive a topical anesthetic on the eye to numb it and prevent it from moving during the laser treatment. During photocoagulation, heat from a high energy laser seals off bleeding in damaged eye tissue.

I will make adjustments to the laser beam before it is aimed into the eye including:

- The amount of energy used
- The size of the "spot" or end of the beam that is directed into the eye
- The pattern applied by the laser beam onto the targeted area

A laser treatment typically lasts at least several minutes, but more time may be required depending on the extent of your eye condition.

During laser treatment, you might experience some discomfort, but you should feel no pain. Right after a treatment, you should be able to resume normal activities. You might have some slight discomfort and blurry vision for a day or two after each laser treatment.

The number of treatments you need will depend on your eye condition and extent of damage. Some people may require three to four different laser sessions at two- to four-week intervals to treat their condition.

Non-Laser Treatments

Steroid Injections

Steroids injected directly into the eye (intraocular steroids) also sometimes are administered in addition to laser treatment to help reduce fluids that accumulate in the retina. Injections are commonly used to treat macular edema as well as macular degeneration

Macular edema (retinal swelling) results from leakage of damaged retinal vessels. Macular edema is common in diabetes, retinal vein occlusions and uveitis. Macular edema damages retinal photoreceptors and leads to loss of vision. Injected directly into the eye, corticosteroids can help reduce swelling and inflammation. You will see floaters for a few days following the injection.

Anti-VEGF Injections

A significant advance has been the development of a new class of drugs now being used to treat wet macular degeneration. The drugs are based on the discovery that a group of proteins in the body, called vascular endothelial growth factor (VEGF), play a significant role in the formation of the abnormal blood vessels that damage the retina in wet macular degeneration. These abnormal blood vessels are called choroidal neovascularization (CNV).

The anti-VEGF drugs are injected directly into the jelly-like substance that fills the back of the eye, which is called the vitreous. Before the injection, drops are used to numb the eye and a speculum may be put in place to hold the eyelids out of the way. While it may seem scary to receive an injection into the eye, most patients find that they experience minimal discomfort. Once inside the eye, the medication diffuses throughout the retina and choroid. It binds strongly to the abnormal VEGF proteins, preventing the proteins from stimulating further unwanted blood vessel growth and leakage. You may see floaters for a few hours following your injection.

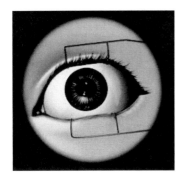 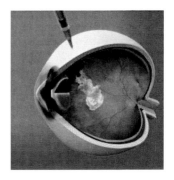

Before injection of an anti-vascular endothelial growth factor (VEGF) drug, the eye is numbed and a speculum may be put in place to keep the eyelids out of the way.

Four anti-VEGF drugs are available on the market for treatment: Avastin, Lucentis, Eyelea and Macugen. Macugen is not as effective as it acts against only one form of the VEGF protein whereas the others target all forms of VEGF.

Lucentis and Eyelea are both FDA approved for use as ocular injections to treat "wet" macular degeneration. Avastin is just as effective at treating "wet" macular degeneration and is used as an off label treatment.

Off label describes use of an FDA-approved drug, treatment, or procedure in a way that has not specifically received U.S. Food and Drug Administration approval. In this case, Avastin is an FDA approved drug for the treatment of colon cancer. However, it is also extremely effective at treating "wet" macular degeneration, but the company that manufactures Avastin has not gone through the process of gaining FDA approval. There are significant costs for the manufacturing company associated with gaining FDA approval for an indication. Those costs are generally passed on to the consumer in the form of higher drug costs.

Avastin is usually my choice for treating "Wet" Macular Degeneration. I have a lot of experience with this drug and have personally seen significant results for my patients. The big advantage that Avastin has over the other drugs is cost. Lucentis and Eyelea cost up to $2000 per treatment, while Avastin costs less than $70.

All three drugs are highly effective. The dramatic and lasting improvements in vision with these drugs is extraordinary.

However, I feel that it is my obligation as a physician to not only choose the best treatment for my patients but to also choose the most cost effective option as to not burden the patient or the health care system.

Typically, injections are given on an every 4-8 week basis (you may require 12 injections a year for two years) until all retinal edema (swelling) has resolved.

Chapter 8

How Long Will I Need To See A Retina Specialist?

Once your treatment plan has been mapped out, you will follow the timeline recommended. If your vision is improving or being well maintained you may simply be scheduled for regular follow up exams. If you are on laser or injection therapy, we will work to find the best frequency for your treatments.

Generally, once you begin seeing a retina specialist, you will continue to see them on some regular basis to be monitored in order to stay on top of any changes in your vision.

Conclusion

Millions of people in North America live with varying degrees of irreversible vision loss because they have an untreatable, degenerative eye disorder. This very large and diverse group of vision disorders affects young and old and people from many cultures, races and ethnicities.

My goal when writing this book is to help you better understand the answers and treatment plan you have been given. But more importantly, we want to help you get your quality of life back so you can continue to do all the activities you so enjoy. Hopefully, this book has given you what you need to proceed with confidence.

Lastly, remember one thing. Saratoga Retina is 100% your advocate. Please do yourself a favor and receive annual eye exams from a Retina Specialist if you have been diagnosed with Diabetes or Macular Degeneration. Both my staff and myself are completely dedicated to improving your vision and therefore your quality of life!

We look forward to serving you. Please call our office at 518-580-0553 or to go our website **www.SaratogaRetina.com** with any questions.

About The Author

Dr. Amjad (Jay) Hammad is the CEO/Owner of Saratoga Vitreo-Retinal Ophthalmology, PLLC and a Clinical Assistant Professor in Ophthalmology specializing in vitreo-retinal surgery and neuro-ophthalmology at the Albany Medical College in Albany, NY.

Jay is originally from Jordan where he was born and raised. He graduated from the College of Medicine at the University of Jordan in the top 5% of his class. Jay came to the states in 1995 and finished a pre-residency clinical/research fellowship in neuro-ophthalmology at Michigan State University in 1997.

Jay completed his ophthalmology residency at the Albany Medical Center in New York in 2000. In his final year, he was awarded the John A. Cetner Excellent Physician Award for outstanding and compassionate care to his patients. He then traveled to San Antonio, Texas for a surgical vitreo-retinal fellowship at the University of Texas Health Science Center at San Antonio.

Jay then returned to his native country for 3 years where he joined the teaching faculty at the University of Jordan and helped teach and improve medical services there. By starting a private medical practice in the city of Amman in Jordan, he helped provide first rate American quality of care to his patients. He facilitated in building and utilizing the country's first ambulatory surgical care center to make modern eye surgery more affordable and convenient to patients and was the personal ophthalmologist to members of the Jordanian Royal Family.

Striving to bring medical care where needed, Jay toured other countries in the Middle East lecturing and examining patients as well as performing surgery.

After returning to the states in 2005, he has joined the clinical academic staff at Albany Medical center as well as starting a private practice in upstate NY. He is currently the CEO of a joint venture with Glens Falls Hospital, The New York Eye Surgical Center, and was elected by his peers to be on the Board of Directors of the New York State Ophthalmology

Society where he chairs the sub-committee on virtual technology.

He is a graduate of the Yale School of Management's Executive MBA – Leadership in Healthcare program, class of 2011 with distinctions in micro and macroeconomics as well as operations management and marketing.

He is both American and Jordanian Board certified in Ophthalmology and was selected recently to be an associate examiner for the American Board of Ophthalmology. He is fluent in both English and Arabic.

Jay and his wife Terry live in Saratoga Springs, NY where they find time to go to the race track and enjoy movies, hiking and table tennis.

His practice Saratoga Vitreo-Retinal is dedicated to helping patients improve their vision in order maintain their quality of life. Dr. Jay has not only been able to achieve great results, but the care and compassion he and his staff have for his patients greatly reduces the stress they can feel during the treatment process.

If you have been diagnosed with Diabetes or Macular Degeneration it is important to receive annual eye exams from a retina specialist. You may make an appointment or ask any questions by calling our office at 518-580-0553. We look forward to serving you.

Appendix A

Glossary

Age Related Macular Degeneration (AMD) - Dry

The macula deteriorates as one ages. Sometimes, the deterioration of the macula, as well as a predilection to risk factors such as heredity, race (lightly pigmented people are more susceptible to the condition than people of darker pigment), smoking, or a high-fat, low-antioxidant diet leads to age-related macular degeneration (AMD).

The dry form of AMD occurs when yellow deposits called drusen form behind the retina. The larger or more prolific these drusen are, the more damage they cause to the pigment epithelial layer of the macula. This layer is directly behind the photoreceptor layer of the macula and provides the sensory cells with an oxygen- and nutrient-rich blood supply. Nearly a quarter of people aged 65 to 74 develop age-related macular degeneration. One out of every three people aged 75 or older is afflicted with the disease. Dry AMD is the most common form of AMD.

Age Related Macular Degeneration (AMD) – Wet

The wet form of AMD occurs when the pigment epithelial layer of the macula, located just behind the layer of cells responsible for central vision, sustains such damage that it breaks. Damage to this thin, mesh-like layer of capillaries may occur because of the presence of drusen or because of fluid accumulating in the sub-retinal space between the two layers.

When the pigment epithelial layer breaks, blood leaks into the photoreceptor layer. In most people, new but very fragile capillaries begin to grow back from the broken membrane, and the condition is further classified as neovascular AMD.

Instead of forming in an organized fashion, these new blood vessels messily make their way into other layers of the macula like unruly tendrils of a vine. These new vessels often break as well, and along with the broken vascular layer, destroy the healthy macula.

Cornea

The clear part of the eye covering the iris and pupil; it lets light into the eye, permitting sight.

Eye Stroke

Eye strokes occur when blockages (occlusions) within veins and arteries cause decreased or distorted vision. Severity of vision loss depends on the extent and location of the problem.

Just as strokes occur in other parts of the body because blood flow is blocked, your eye also may suffer damage when vital structures such as the retina and optic nerve are cut off from nutrients and oxygen flowing through your blood.

Besides having an eye exam to detect signs of an eye occlusion, you'll also need your family doctor or internal medicine physician to evaluate you for high blood pressure, artery disease or heart problems that may be responsible for the blockage.

If a blockage is found, the type of eye occlusion you have is categorized by its location.

Floaters

Eye floaters are those tiny spots, specks, flecks and "cobwebs" that drift aimlessly around in your field of vision. While annoying, ordinary eye floaters and spots are very common and usually aren't cause for alarm. Floaters and spots typically appear when tiny pieces of the eye's gel-like vitreous break loose within the inner back portion of the eye.

When we are born and throughout our youth, the vitreous has a gel-like consistency. But as we age, the vitreous begins to dissolve and liquefy to create a watery center. Some undissolved gel particles occasionally will float around in the more liquid center of the vitreous. These particles can take on many shapes and sizes to become what we refer to as "floaters."

You'll notice that these types of spots and floaters are particularly pronounced when you peer at a bright, clear sky or a white computer screen. But you can't actually see tiny bits of debris floating loose within your eye. Instead, shadows from these floaters are cast on the retina as light passes through the eye, and those shadows are what you see.

You'll also notice that these specks never seem to stay still when you try to focus on them. Floaters and spots move when your eye moves, creating the impression that they are "drifting."

Fluorescein angiography

An imaging test that involves first injecting fluorescent yellow-green dye into the veins. When the dye reaches interior regions of the eye, it provides opportunity for high contrast photography or other imaging of blood vessels.

Fluorescein angiography particularly is useful in diagnosing conditions such as age-related macular degeneration, which in advanced forms can be characterized by abnormal growth of blood vessels in the retina.

Ischemia

Poor blood flow. Obstructions such as clots in veins and arteries can block blood flow, depriving tissue of oxygen and nutrients. These blockages also can cause "eye strokes" and sudden vision loss.

Laser photocoagulation

Procedure in which a surgeon uses a laser to coagulate tissue, usually to seal leaking blood vessels and destroy new ones in diseases like macular degeneration and diabetic retinopathy.

Macula

At the back of the eye, directly in line with the pupil, is an area of the retina called the macula. In the center of the macula is an indentation called the fovea that is packed with cones; cells that require high levels of light in order to function.

As light enters the eye through the pupil, it is concentrated into the area of the macula and the fovea. Because of the cones that comprise the macula, central vision is crisp, clear, detailed and in color.

The macula, an area just 5mm in diameter (roughly the thickness of a fingernail), is responsible for the vision that is necessary for many daily activities. Any condition that impairs this area will adversely affect central vision and the ability to carry out many activities that are important to daily life.

Macular edema
Swelling of the central portion of the retina (macula), due to buildup of fluid leaking from retinal blood vessels. Causes temporary or permanent vision loss if untreated.

Macular Hole
A macular hole, also known as a macular cyst, is a small hole formed in the macula due to tension on the surface of the retina due to shrinking vitreous. With age, the structures of the eye change. This is true of the gel-like fluid vitreous, which fills the area between the lens and the retina. Over time, its composition changes; its fibers begin to clump together and

shrink away from the retina.

This is a natural occurrence and usually has no negative effects. Occasionally though, in areas where it is firmly adhered to the retina, it will pull the retina with it. The shrinking vitreous can cause a macular hole when it pulls on the macula. The macular hole will cause distortion in the central line of vision.

Reading will become difficult because lines will appear wavy. If the shrinking vitreous has caused a hole that is the full thickness of the macula, there will be an area of central vision that will simply be missing.

Microaneurysm
A weakened area in the walls of tiny blood vessels. In diabetic retinopathy, microaneurysms can occur in the retina from damage related to abnormally high blood sugar levels. As microaneurysms in tiny blood vessels (capillaries) expand, ruptures can result. These ruptures lead to hampered blood

flow as well as swelling and leakage that sometimes cause scarring, blind spots and blindness.

Neovascularization

Abnormal growth of new blood vessels, such as in an excessive amount, or in tissue that normally does not contain them, or of a different kind than is usual in that tissue.

Ophthalmologist

An ophthalmologist (MD or DO) is a medical or osteopathic doctor who specializes in the eye. They perform eye exams, diagnose and treat disease, prescribe medication, and perform surgery. They may also write prescriptions for eyeglasses, and contact lenses.

Ophthalmologists complete four years of medical school, one year of internship, and a minimum of three years of residency in ophthalmology.

Optic Nerve

At the back of the eye, a few millimeters toward the nose from center, is the optic nerve. The optic nerve connects the eye to the brain and relays information about sight. Photoreceptors receive light waves and instantly convert the information to electrical impulses.

These electric signals travel from cell to cell along microscopic nerve fibers, being processed and analyzed along the way. Eventually, the nerve fibers and their information, in the form of electrical impulses, converge. Thousands of signals then travel the length of the optic nerve to the brain, where they are processed and understood.

Optometrist

An optometrist (OD) is an eye doctor who examines eyes for both vision and health problems, and corrects refractive error by prescribing eyeglasses and contact lenses. Optometrists diagnose and treat eye problems and diseases, and prescribe many ophthalmic medications and may participate in your pre-

and postoperative care if you have eye surgery but do not perform surgery themselves.

Some optometrists provide low vision rehabilitation and vision therapy. An optometrist must complete four years of post-graduate optometry school, and some complete a residency with advanced study in a specific area of eye care.

Photoreceptors

Light-sensitive cells found in the retina. Photoreceptors in the human retina are classified as cones and rods. Cones are located in the central retina (the fovea) and control color vision. Rods are located outside the fovea and control black/white vision in low-light conditions.

Retina

The sensory membrane that lines the back of the eye. Cells in the retina called photoreceptors transform light energy into electrical signals that are transmitted to the brain by way of the optic nerve.

Retina Specialist

Retina specialists are highly trained Ophthalmologists. They must complete medical school and specialized training as an ophthalmologist, and then pursue additional vitreo-retinal training. The full breadth of training for a retina specialist includes:

• Undergraduate College – 4 years

• Medical School - 4 years

• Internship - 1 year

• Ophthalmology Residency - 3 years

• Retina-Vitreous Fellowship - 2 years

Retinopathy

Any change in the retina due to disease or damage is called a retinopathy. Some retinopathies are the result of underlying disease, such as diabetes or hypertension. Other retinopathies occur because of exposure to a toxin or an adverse reaction to something in the environment. Certain drugs, extreme bright sunlight, and even high altitude can cause retinopathy.

Retinopathy may result in blurred vision or vision loss, due to the abnormal growth of capillaries in the retina and any leaking or hemorrhaging that occurs. In many cases, treatment of the underlying disease improves vision.

Vitreous body

Part of the eye between the lens and the retina, containing a clear jelly, sometimes also called the vitreous humor.

Appendix B

Instructions for administering eye drops:

Effective Way To Put Drops In Your Eye

1. Create a pocket by pulling down on your lower lid
2. Put one drop of the medication in the lower lid pocket
3. Gently close BOTH eyes, Do not squeeze or blink
4. Count to 30, allowing the medication to be absorbed
5. If more than one medication has been prescribed, wait at least 5 minutes and follow steps 1-4.

Dr. Amjad Hammad (Dr. Jay)

Saratoga Vitreo-Retinal Ophthalmology
465 Maple Avenue
Unit B
Saratoga Springs, New York 12866

Phone: 518-580-0553

www.SaratogaRetina.com